The E.C.G. Made Easy

The E.C.G. Made Easy

John R. Hampton D.M., D.Phil., F.R.C.P.

Reader in Medicine
Nottingham University

CHURCHILL LIVINGSTONE
EDINBURGH LONDON AND NEW YORK
1973

CHURCHILL LIVINGSTONE
Medical Division of Longman Group Limited

Distributed in the United States of America by
Longman Inc., 19 West 44th Street, New York, N.Y. 10036,
and by associated companies, branches and representatives
throughout the world.

First published 1973
Reprinted 1975
Reprinted 1976
Reprinted 1977

ISBN 0 443 01036 6

Printed in Hong Kong by
Wing King Tong Co Ltd

PREFACE

About half the people who are going to die from a heart attack do so within two hours of the onset of symptoms, and any reduction in the mortality from heart attacks depends on the rapid identification of abnormal cardiac rhythms. A working knowledge of the electrocardiogram is therefore essential to all those who may be faced with patients with heart attacks, and this little book is intended for general practitioners, medical students, and nurses in coronary and intensive care units.

Increasing interest in cardiac arrhythmias has brought greater understanding of the physiology underlying normal and abnormal electrocardiograms, and also a greater complexity of books on the subject. This book makes no pretensions of completeness, only of simplicity. Most people drive cars without understanding much of what goes on under the bonnet, and most people can make use of an electrocardiogram without getting too involved in its complexities. In other words, this book is for gardeners and not for botanists. It is not concerned with the management of patients with heart disease, but as a practitioner may wish to carry it tucked into his ECG recorder, the most basic management of arrhythmias has been included in the flow diagram at the end of chapter 2.

I am grateful to Professor J. R. A. Mitchell, Dr D. C. Banks, and Dr G. K. Morris for their suggestions and criticism, and to Mrs M. Cameron and Mr G. Lyth for help with the illustrations.

Department of Medicine,
Nottingham University   JOHN HAMPTON

CONTENTS

Chapter 1

WHAT THE E.C.G. IS ABOUT

Principles
1 The E.C.G. is easy to understand.
2 Most abnormalities of the E.C.G. are amenable to reason.

The electricity of the heart
The contraction of any muscle is associated with electrical changes called 'depolarisation', and these changes can be detected by electrodes attached to the surface of the body. Since all muscular contraction will be detected the electrical changes associated with contraction of the heart muscle will only be clear if the patient is fully relaxed and no skeletal muscles are contracting.

Although the heart has four chambers, from the electrical point of view it can be thought of as having only two, for the two atria contract together and then the two ventricles contract together.

The muscle mass of the atria is relatively small and the electrical change accompanying their contraction is therefore small. Contraction of the atria causes the E.C.G. wave called 'P'. Since the ventricular mass is large there is a large deflection of the E.C.G. when the

ventricles contract and this is called the 'QRS' complex.
The 'T' wave of the E.C.G. is caused by the return of
this ventricular mass to the resting electrical state
(repolarisation).

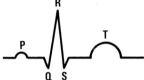

Definitions

The different parts of the QRS complex are arbitrarily
labelled. If the first deflection is downwards, it is
called a Q wave.

A deflection upwards is called an R wave,

—whether it is preceded by a Q or not.

Any deflection below the baseline following an R
wave is called an S wave,

—whether there has been a preceding Q or not.

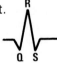

The wiring diagram of the heart

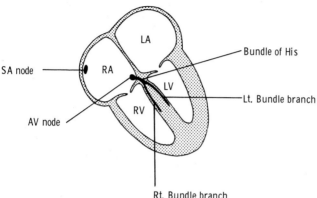

The electrical discharge for each cardiac cycle starts in a special area of the right atrium called the 'sino-atrial' (SA) node. Depolarisation then spreads through the atrial muscle fibres. There is a delay while depolarisation spreads through another special area in the atrium, the atrioventricular node (also called the 'AV node', or sometimes just 'the node'.) Thereafter conduction is very rapid down specialised conduction tissue: first a single pathway, the 'bundle of His' and then this divides in the septum between the ventricles into right and left bundle branches. The left bundle branch itself divides into two. Within the mass of ventricular muscle conduction spreads rapidly through specialised fibres.

Times and speeds

It is a fundamental principle of E.C.G. machines that they all run at a standard rate and they use paper with standard squares. Each large square is equivalent to 0·2 seconds, so there are five large squares per second, and 300 per minute. So an E.C.G. event, such as a QRS complex, occurring once per large square is occurring at a rate of 300 per minute. The heart rate can be calculated rapidly by remembering this sequence: If the R—R interval is:

1 large square, the rate is 300 per minute
2 ,, ,, ,, ,, ,, 150 ,, ,,
3 ,, ,, ,, ,, ,, 100 ,, ,,
4 ,, ,, ,, ,, ,, 75 ,, ,,
5 ,, ,, ,, ,, ,, 60 ,, ,,
6 ,, ,, ,, ,, ,, 50 ,, ,,

Just as the length of paper between R waves gives the heart rate, so the distance between the different parts of the P—QRS—T complex shows the time taken for conduction to occur through different parts of the heart.

PR INTERVAL

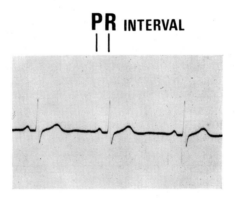

The PR interval is the time taken for excitation to spread from the SA node, through the atrial muscle and the AV node, down the bundle of His and into the ventricular muscle. Most of the time is taken up by delay in the AV node. The normal PR interval is 0·12 to 0·2 seconds (3 to 5 small squares). If the PR interval is very short, either the atria have been depolarised from close to the AV node, or there is an abnormality of conduction from the atria to the ventricles.

The duration of the QRS complex shows how long excitation takes to spread through the ventricles. The QRS duration is normally 0·12 seconds (three small squares) or less but any abnormality of conduction takes longer, and causes widened QRS complexes.

Recording an E.C.G.

The purpose of recording the E.C.G. from several leads is to look at the heart from several different directions. The limb leads are attached to metal plates, which are held in contact by rubber straps. Good contact will only be achieved if electrode jelly is rubbed into the skin under the plates. The limb leads are marked 'RA, LA, LL, and RL' for the right and left arms and legs. It is not necessary to remember the internal connections of the machine—it is much easier to be certain that the leads are properly attached.

The 12-lead E.C.G.
It is, however, useful to remember the directions from which the various leads 'look at' the heart. The six 'standard' leads can be thought of as looking at the heart in a vertical plane (that is, from the sides or the feet).

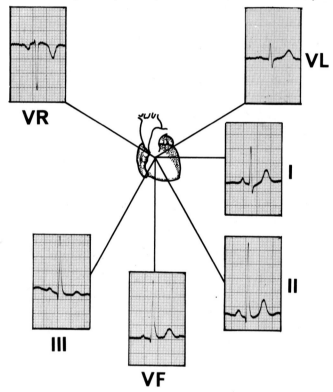

Thus leads I, II and VL look at the left lateral surface of the heart, III and VF at the inferior surface, and VR looks at the atria.

The V lead is fixed in different positions by means of a suction cup: again the skin must be rubbed with electrode jelly, but it is essential that the jellied areas should not touch. The leads look directly at the heart in a horizontal plane (that is, from the front).

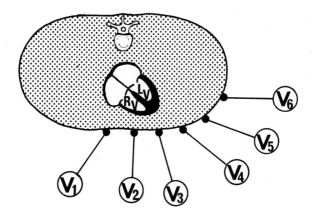

Thus leads V1 and V2 look at the right ventricle, V3 and V4 look at the septum between the ventricles and the anterior wall of the left ventricle, and V5 and V6 look at the anterior and lateral walls of the left ventricle.

The V lead positions are in the fourth and fifth rib spaces:

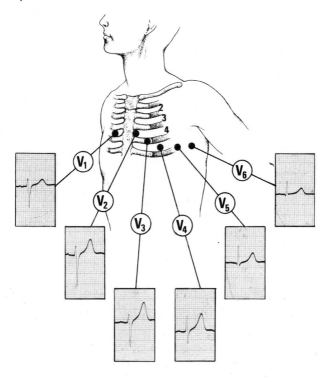

The size of the E.C.G. deflection will depend on the mass of muscle in the heart, and may be reduced if the heart is 'insulated' by a pericardial effusion. It is essential therefore that at the beginning of each record the 1 mV standard should be recorded: if the needle does not move one centimetre up the paper, the sensitivity control must be adjusted until it does.

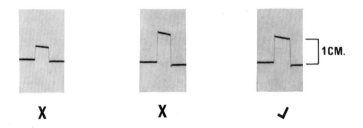

So, when making a recording:

1 The patient must lie down and relax. (Prevent muscle tremor)
2 Connect up the limb leads, making certain that they are applied to the correct limb.
3 Record the sensitivity.
4 Record the six standard leads—three or four complexes are sufficient for each.
5 Record the six V leads.

THE SHAPE OF THE QRS COMPLEX

(a) The QRS in the limb leads

The E.C.G. machine is arranged so that when a depolarisation wave spreads towards an electrode the needle moves upwards and when it spreads away from the electrode the needle moves downwards.

The deflection of the QRS complex thus shows the direction in which the wave of depolarisation is spreading. If it is predominantly upwards (that is, the R wave is greater than the S wave), the depolarisation is moving towards that electrode.

9

If predominantly downwards (S greater than R), the depolarisation is moving away.

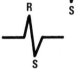

When the depolarisation wave is moving at right angles to the electrode then R and S waves are equal.

Q waves have a special significance which we shall discuss later.

AVR and II look at the heart from opposite directions. Seen from the front, the depolarising wave normally spreads down from 11 o'clock to 5 o'clock so the deflections in AVR are normally mainly downwards and in II mainly upwards.

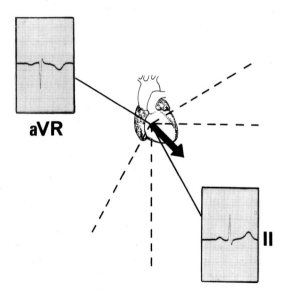

The average direction of spread of the depolarisation wave as seen from the front is called the *cardiac axis* and it is useful to decide whether this axis is in a normal direction or not. The axis can be deduced from leads I, II and III.

The normal 11 o'clock—5 o'clock axis means that the depolarising wave is spreading towards leads I, II and III and is therefore associated with a predominantly upward deflection in all; the deflection will be greater in II than I or III.

NORMAL AXIS

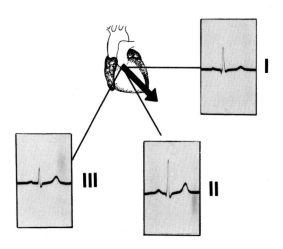

If the right ventricle becomes hypertrophied the axis will swing towards the right: the deflection in I becomes negative and the deflection in III will become positive. This is called *right axis deviation*, and it is associated mainly with pulmonary conditions that put a strain on the right side of the heart, and with congenital heart disorders.

RIGHT AXIS DEVIATION

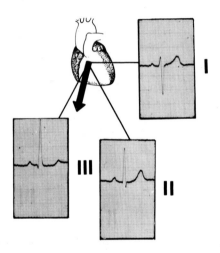

When the left ventricle becomes hypertrophied the axis may swing to the left, so that the QRS becomes predominantly negative in III. *Left axis deviation* is not significant until the QRS deflection is also predominantly negative in II:

LEFT AXIS DEVIATION

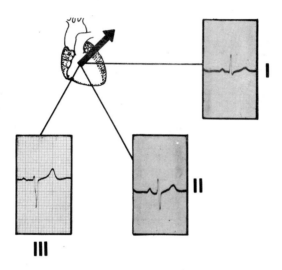

In the case of left axis deviation the problem is usually due to a conduction defect rather than to the increased bulk of left ventricular muscle, but the principle is the same.

Right and left axis deviation of themselves are seldom significant—minor degrees occur respectively in long, thin, and short, fat individuals—but their presence should alert you to look for other signs of right and left ventricular hypertrophy, which we shall discuss in chapter 3.

(b) The QRS in the V leads

The shape of the QRS complex in the chest (V) leads is determined by two things.

1   The septum between the ventricles is depolarised first, and the depolarisation wave spreads across the septum from left to right.

2   In the normal heart there is more muscle in the wall of the left ventricle than in the right ventricle, and the left ventricle therefore exerts more influence on the E.C.G. pattern than the right ventricle.

The leads V1 and V2 are 'looking at' the right ventricle. Lead V3 and V4 look at the septum and V5 and V6 at the left ventricle. In a right ventricular lead the deflection is first upwards (R wave) as the septum is depolarised;

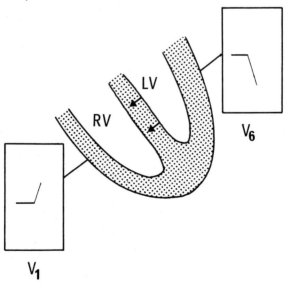

and then downwards (S wave) as the main muscle
mass is depolarised;

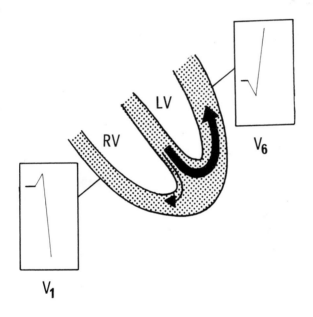

the bigger LV (in which depolarisation is spreading
away) outweighing the effects of the smaller RV (in
which depolarisation is spreading towards the
electrode).

In a left ventricular lead the opposite pattern is seen.
There is a small downward deflection ('septal Q wave')
as the septum is depolarised, and then an upward
deflection (R wave) as the ventricular muscle is
depolarised. When the whole of the myocardium is
depolarised the E.C.G. returns to the baseline.

Things to remember

1   The E.C.G. results from electrical changes associated with contraction first of the atria and then of the ventricles.
2   Atrial contraction causes the P wave.
3   Ventricular contraction causes the QRS complex. If the first deflection is down it is a Q. If the first deflection is up it is an R. A downwards deflection after an R is an S.

4   When the depolarisation wave spreads towards an electrode the deflection is upwards.
5   The direction of the QRS in leads I, II and III depends on the cardiac axis.
6   The V leads provide specific information about the right and left ventricles.

Chapter 2

THE RHYTHM OF THE HEART

When interpreting an E.C.G. first identify the rhythm.

Principles
1 The E.C.G. is easy to understand.
2 Abnormalities of cardiac rhythm are particularly easy to work out, and the key is the P wave.

When attempting to analyse a cardiac rhythm remember:
(a) atrial contraction is associated with the E.C.G. P wave,
(b) ventricular contraction is associated with the E.C.G. QRS complex,
(c) atrial contraction normally precedes ventricular contraction, and there is normally one atrial contraction per ventricular contraction. (i.e. there should be as many P waves as there are QRS complexes.)

THE INTRINSIC RHYTHMICITY OF THE HEART
Most parts of the heart will depolarise spontaneously and rhythmically, and the rate of contraction of the

ventricles will be controlled by the part of the heart that is depolarising most frequently. The sino-atrial (SA) node normally has the highest frequency of discharge and therefore the rate of contraction of the ventricles will follow that of the SA node. This normal state of affairs is called *sinus rhythm.*

The rate of discharge of the SA node is influenced by the vagal nerve, and reflexes originating in the lung affect the heart rate. Changes in rate associated with respiration are normally seen in young people, and this is called *sinus arrhythmia.*

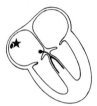

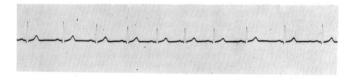

Note: One P wave per QRS complex.
      Constant PR interval.
      Progressive beat-to-beat change in R–R interval.

A slow sinus rhythm (sinus bradycardia) is associated with athletic training, fainting attacks, hypothermia, myxoedema, and it is often seen immediately after a heart attack. A fast sinus rhythm (sinus tachycardia) is associated with exercise, fear, pain, haemorrhage, and thyrotoxicosis.

ABNORMALITIES IN THE CONNECTIONS BETWEEN THE ATRIA AND THE VENTRICLES

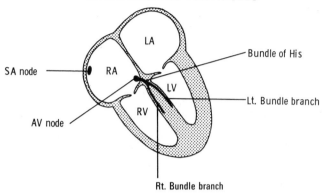

The time taken by the spread of depolarisation from the SA node to the ventricular muscle is shown by the PR interval (chapter 1) and is not normally greater than 0·2 seconds (one large square). Interference with the conduction process causes the E.C.G. phenomenon called 'heart block'.

If each wave of depolarisation that originates in the SA node is conducted to the ventricles but there is delay somewhere along the conduction pathway, then the PR interval is prolonged and this is called *first degree heart block.*

.36 SECS.

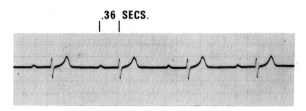

Note: One P wave per QRS complex.
       PR interval 0·36 seconds.

First degree heart block is not of itself important, but it may be a sign of coronary artery disease, acute rheumatic carditis, digitalis toxicity or electrolyte disturbances.

Sometimes excitation completely fails to pass through the AV node or the bundle of His. When this occurs intermittently *second degree heart block* is said to exist. There are three variations of this:

(a) Most beats are conducted with a normal PR interval, but occasionally there is an atrial contraction without a subsequent ventricular contraction. This is called the 'Mobitz type 2' phenomenon.

P

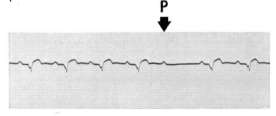

Note : PR interval of the conducted beats is constant (in this case, prolonged to 0·24 seconds, indicating a first degree heart block). One P wave is not followed by a QRS complex and here 'second degree' block is occurring.

(b) There may be progressive lengthening of the PR interval and then failure of conduction of an atrial beat, followed by a conducted beat with a short PR interval and then a repetition of this cycle. This is the 'Wenkebach phenomenon'.

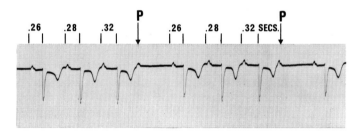

Note: Progressive lengthening of PR interval.
      One non-conducted beat.
      Next conducted beat has a shorter PR interval.

(c)   There may be alternate conducted and non-
      conducted atrial beats (or one conducted atrial
      beat and then two non-conducted beats), giving
      twice (or three times) as many P waves as QRS
      complexes. This is called '2 to 1' (or '3 to 1')
      conduction.

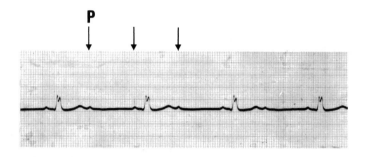

Note: Two P waves per QRS complex.
      Normal, and constant, PR interval in the
      conducted beats.
      In this example the QRS is notched indicating
      an abnormality of conduction also exists within
      the ventricles.

The Rhythm of the Heart

It is important to remember with this as with any other rhythm, that a P wave may only show itself as a distortion of a T wave.

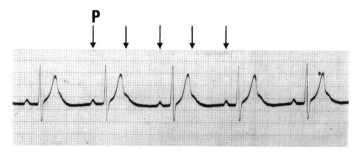

Note: P wave in the T wave can be identified because of its regularity.

The causes of second degree heart block are the same as those of first degree block. In patients with heart attacks the Wenkebach phenomenon is usually benign, but Mobitz type 2 block and 2 to 1 block may herald complete, or third degree, heart block.

Complete heart block (third degree block) is said to occur when atrial contraction is normal but no beats are conducted to the ventricles. When this occurs the ventricles are excited by a slow 'escape mechanism' (see below), with a depolarising focus within the ventricular muscle.

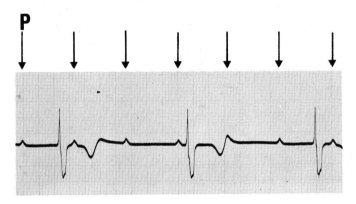

Note: P wave rate 90 per minute.
      QRS rate 36 per minute.
      No relation between P and QRS.
      Abnormal shaped QRS complexes because of abnormal spread of depolarisation from ventricular focus.

Complete heart block may occur as an acute phenomenon in patients with heart attacks (when it is usually transient) or it may be a chronic state, usually due to fibrosis around the bundle of His.

'ESCAPE RHYTHMS'—THE SLOW RHYTHMS

If the SA node slows markedly, or ceases to discharge altogether, the region of the heart with the next highest intrinsic rate of discharge will take over and control the rate of ventricular contraction. The heart therefore has a protective mechanism which keeps it going if something goes wrong with part of its depolarising mechanism. The order of frequency of discharge is the same as the order in which the normal depolarisation wave spreads through the heart:

The SA node depolarises most often
then atrial muscle
then the region around the AV node
then ventricular muscle.

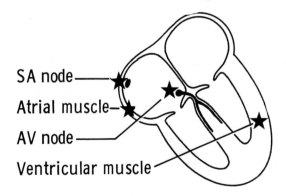

SA node
Atrial muscle
AV node
Ventricular muscle

Escape rhythms are therefore mainly *slow*, and together with sinus bradycardia and heart block they constitute the 'brady-arrhythmias'. Escape rhythms are not primary disorders, but are the response to problems higher in the conducting pathway: they are commonly

25

seen in the acute phase of a heart attack, often associated with sinus bradycardia. It is useful to consider them before the more dramatic fast arrhythmias because they show the type of E.C.G. pattern that is associated with rhythms originating in different parts of the heart.

The Rhythm of the Heart

If the SA node slows down and a focus in the atrium takes over control of the heart, the rhythm is described as *'atrial escape'*. Atrial escape beats can occur singly.

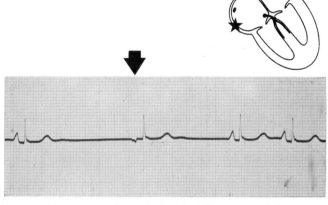

Note: After one sinus beat the SA node fails to depolarise. After a delay an abnormal P wave is seen because excitation of the atrium has begun somewhere away from the SA node. The abnormal P wave is followed by a normal QRS, because excitation has spread normally down the His Bundle. The third and fourth beats show a return to sinus rhythm.

Atrial escape rhythms may be sustained, and when this happens depolarisation may begin in a different part of the atrium each time, giving rise to continuously changing P wave shapes and changes in the PR interval. This phenomenon is called a 'wandering atrial pacemaker'.

If the region around the AV node takes over, the rhythm is called *nodal*, or more properly, *junctional*.

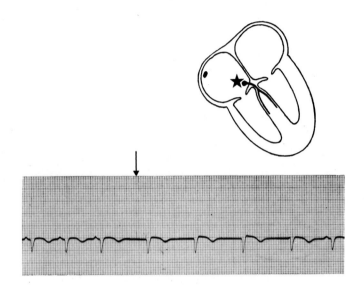

Note: Sinus rate 100 per minute; junctional escape (following arrow) at 70 per minute.
   No P waves in junctional beats (either no atrial contraction, or P wave lost in QRS).
   Normal QRS.

Ventricular escape most commonly occurs when conduction between the atria and ventricles is interrupted, and complete heart block is the classical ventricular escape rhythm.

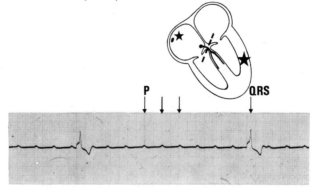

Note: Regular P waves (normal atrial conduction).
P wave rate 145 per minute.
Regular QRS, but complexes highly abnormal because of abnormal conduction through ventricular muscle. QRS (ventricular escape) rate 15 per minute.
No relation between P waves and QRS complexes.

EXTRASYSTOLES

Any part of the heart can depolarise earlier than it should, and the accompanying heart beat is called an extrasystole. The term 'ectopic' is sometimes used to indicate that conduction originated in an abnormal place; 'premature contraction' is also used.

The E.C.G. appearance of an extrasystole arising in the atrial muscle, the junctional or nodal region, or in the ventricular muscle, is the same as that of the

29

corresponding 'escape' beat—the difference is that an extrasystole comes early, and an escape beat comes late.

Extrasystoles are conveniently divided into those arising in the atria and junctional area ('supraventricular') and those arising in the ventricles ('ventricular').

Supraventricular

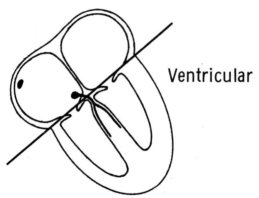

Ventricular

It is important to differentiate between the two, as supraventricular extrasystoles are seldom of importance, while ventricular extrasystoles may well be.

The simplest way of differentiating supraventricular from ventricular extrasystoles is that in the former the QRS complex looks very similar to that following a normal sinus beat, while ventricular extrasystoles look different.

The Rhythm of the Heart

SINUS

JUNCTIONAL }
ATRIAL }
SUPRAVENTRICULAR
EXTRASYSTOLES

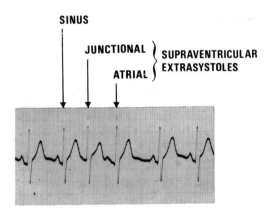

Note: This record shows sinus rhythm with junctional
and atrial extrasystoles.
Sinus, junctional and atrial beats have identical
QRS complexes—conduction in and beyond
the bundle of His is normal.
Junctional extrasystole has no P wave.
Atrial extrasystole has an abnormal shaped P
wave.

VENTRICULAR

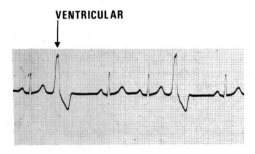

Note: Ventricular extrasystole has abnormal QRS
shape.

It may, however, not be as easy as this, particularly if a beat of supraventricular origin is conducted abnormally to the ventricles (see bundle branch block—chapter 3). It is best to get in the habit of asking five questions every time:

1   Does the early QRS complex follow an early P wave? If it does, it must be an atrial extrasystole.

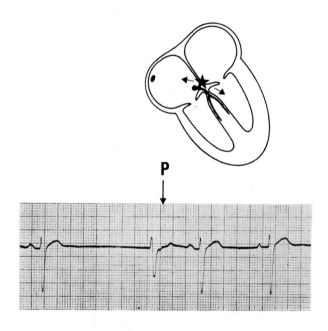

Note: A late (escape) nodal beat with a normal QRS and a P wave between the QRS and the T wave.

2   Can a P wave be seen anywhere? A junctional
    extrasystole may cause the appearance of a P
    wave very close to, and even after, the QRS
    complex because it is conducted both to the atria
    and to the ventricles.
3   Is the QRS complex the same shape (i.e. has it the
    same initial direction of deflection as the normal
    beat, and is it the same duration)? Supra-
    ventricular beats look the same, ventricular beats
    look different.
4   Is the T wave the same way up as in the normal
    beat? Supraventricular—same. Ventricular—
    different.
5   Does the next P wave after the extrasystole appear
    at an expected time? In both supraventricular and
    ventricular extrasystoles there is a ('compensatory')
    pause before the next heart beat, but a supra-
    ventricular extrasystole usually upsets the normal
    periodicity of the SA node, so that the next SA
    node discharge (and P wave) comes late.

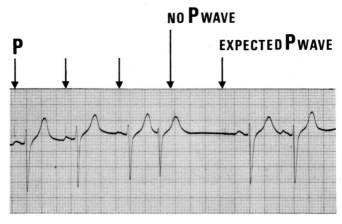

NO **P** WAVE

P

EXPECTED **P** WAVE

A ventricular extrasystole, on the other hand, usually does not affect the SA node, so the next P wave appears at a predicted time.

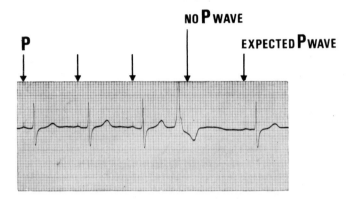

Sometimes some of the answers to these questions will suggest the extrasystole is supraventricular, and some will suggest it is ventricular—when this happens, the extrasystole must be considered to be the type indicated by the majority of the answers.

THE TACHYCARDIAS—THE FAST RHYTHMS

Foci in the atria, the junctional (AV nodal) region, and ventricles may fire repeatedly, causing a sustained tachycardia. The same criteria as above can be used to decide the origin of the arrhythmia, and as before the most important thing is to try to identify a P wave.

(a) Supraventricular tachycardias
1 Atrial tachycardia (abnormal focus in the atrium). In atrial tachycardia the atria contract faster than 160

per minute. The ventricles cannot follow atrial rates above about 200 per minute, and atrio-ventricular block occurs. When the atrial rate is above 250, and there is no flat baseline between P waves, *atrial flutter* is present.

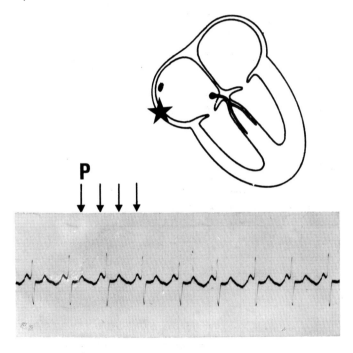

Note: P wave rate 250 per minute.
QRS rate 125 per minute.
QRS complexes regular and of a normal-looking configuration.

Carotid sinus pressure may have a useful therapeutic effect on supraventricular tachycardias, and is always worth trying as it may make the nature of the arrhythmia more obvious.

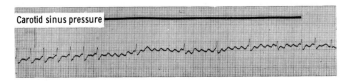

In this case, carotid sinus pressure has increased the block between atria and ventricles, and has revealed that the underlying rhythm is atrial flutter.

2 Junctional ('nodal') tachycardia. If the area around the AV node depolarises frequently, the P waves may be seen very close to the QRS (as with the corresponding extrasystoles) or may not be seen at all. The QRS complex is of normal shape because, as with the other supraventricular arrhythmias, the ventricles are activated down the bundle of His in the normal way.

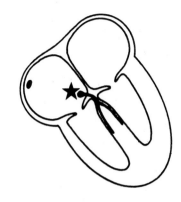

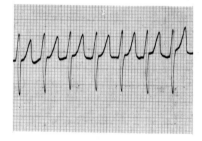

Note: No P wave.
Normal QRS complexes.
QRS complexes completely regular.

(b) Ventricular tachycardias

If a focus in the ventricular muscle depolarises at a high frequency (causing, in effect, rapidly repeated ventricular extrasystoles) the rhythm is called ventricular tachycardia. Excitation has to spread by an abnormal path through the ventricular muscle, and the QRS complex is wide and abnormal.

37

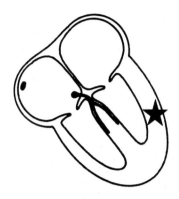

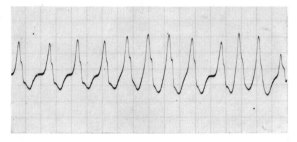

Note: No P waves.
Wide QRS complexes.
QRS complexes slightly irregular and vary
slightly in shape.

FIBRILLATION

All the arrhythmias so far discussed have involved
the synchronous contraction of all the muscle fibres
of the atria or of the ventricles, albeit at abnormal
speeds. When individual muscle fibres contract
independently they are said to be 'fibrillating'.
Fibrillation can occur in the atrial or ventricular muscle.

The Rhythm of the Heart

When the atrial muscle fibres contract independently there are no P waves on the E.C.G. but only an irregular line. At times there may be 'flutter'-like waves for 2 or 3 seconds. The AV node is continuously bombarded with depolarisation waves of varying strength, and depolarisation spreads at irregular intervals down the bundle of His. The ventricles therefore contract irregularly, but because conduction into and through the ventricles is by the normal route, the QRS complex is a normal shape.

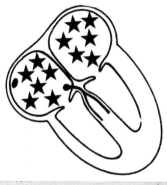

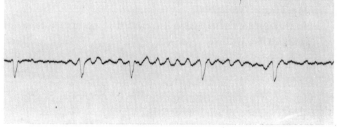

Note: No P waves—irregular baseline.
Irregular QRS complexes.
Normal shaped QRS.

Ventricular fibrillation

When the ventricular muscle fibres contract independently no QRS complex can be identified and the E.C.G. is totally disorganised.

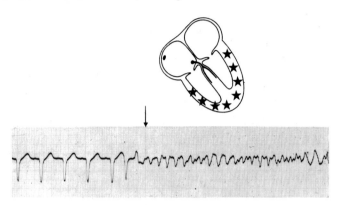

As the patient will usually have lost consciousness by the time you have realised that it is not just due to a loose connection, the diagnosis is easy.

Things to remember

1 Most parts of the heart are capable of spontaneous depolarisation.
2 Heart block results from delay in, or interruption of, the normal conducting pathway.
3 Escape rhythms are slow, and are protective.
4 Occasional early depolarisation of any part of the heart causes an extrasystole.
5 Frequent depolarisation of any part of the heart causes a tachycardia.
6 Asynchronous contraction of muscle fibres in the atria or ventricles is called fibrillation.

7   Apart from the rate, the E.C.G. pattern of an
    escape rhythm, an extrasystole, and a tachycardia
    arising in any one part of the heart is the same.
8   All supraventricular rhythms have normal QRS
    complexes provided there is no bundle branch
    block (chapter 3).

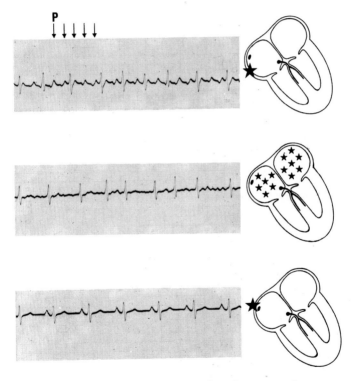

Note: These three records were taken from a patient
      being treated for atrial flutter. During treatment

he developed transient atrial fibrillation before converting to sinus rhythm.
First record shows P waves at 260 per minute.
Second record shows no P waves.
Third record shows P waves at 75 per minute.
In each record QRS appearance is the same.

Recognising E.C.G. abnormalities is to a large extent like recognising an elephant—once seen, never forgotten. However, in cases of difficulty it is helpful to ask the following questions, referring to Table 1.
(a) Is the abnormality occasional or sustained?
(b) Are there any P waves?
(c) Are there as many QRS complexes as P waves?
(d) Are the ventricles contracting regularly or irregularly?
(e) Is the QRS complex a normal shape?
(f) What is the ventricular rate?

Table 1 also shows the most basic methods for treating arrhythmias, using only lignocaine, atropine and digoxin. It is worth remembering that many abnormalities of cardiac rhythm can be induced by too much Digoxin, and if a patient on Digoxin develops an arrhythmias the first thing to do is to stop this drug.

Table 1

Abnormality	P wave	P:QRS ratio	QRS regularity	QRS shape	QRS rate	Rhythm	First line treatment
Occasional	(i.e. extrasystoles)			Normal		Supraventricular	Nothing
				Abnormal		Ventricular	Nothing or lignocaine
Sustained	Present	P's = QRS's	Regular	Normal	Normal	Sinus rhythm	Nothing
					180 +	Atrial tachycardia	Digoxin
			Slightly irregular	Normal	Normal	Sinus arrhythmia	Nothing
					Slow	Atrial escape	Atropine
		More P's than QRS's	Regular	Normal	Fast	Atrial tachycardia with block	Digoxin
					Slow	2° Heart block	Nothing
				Abnormal	Slow	Complete heart block	Hospital
	Absent		Regular	Normal	Fast	Nodal tachycardia	Digoxin
					Slow	Nodal escape	Atropine
				Abnormal	Fast	Nodal tachycardia with bundle branch block	Hospital
			Slightly irregular	Abnormal	Fast	Ventricular tachycardia	Lignocaine then hospital
			Very irregular	Normal	Any speed	Atrial fibrillation	Digoxin
			QRS absent			Ventricular fibrillation or standstill	Cardiac massage

Chapter 3

ABNORMALITIES OF THE P, QRS, AND T WAVES

When interpreting an E.C.G., identify the rhythm first. Then ask the following questions—always in the same sequence:
1   Are there any abnormalities of the P wave?
2   What is the cardiac axis? (Look at the QRS in leads I, II, III—and at chapter 1 if necessary.)
3   Is the QRS of normal duration?
4   Are there any other abnormalities in the QRS— particularly in height, and in the presence of Q waves?
5   Is the ST segment raised or depressed?
6   Is the T wave normal?

Principles
1   The E.C.G. is easy to understand.
2   The P wave can only be normal, unusually tall, or unusually broad.
3   The QRS complex can only have three abnormalities—it can be too broad, too tall, and it may contain an abnormal Q wave.
4   The ST segment can only be normal, elevated, or depressed.

5   The T wave can only be the right way up or the wrong way up.

ABNORMALITIES OF THE P WAVE

Apart from alterations of the shape of the P wave associated with rhythm changes, there are only two important abnormalities:

1   Anything that causes the right atrium to become hypertrophied (tricuspid valve stenosis, or pulmonary hypertension) causes the P to become peaked.

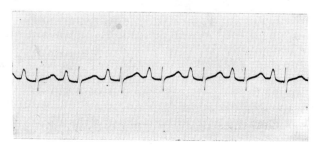

2   Left atrial hypertrophy (usually due to mitral stenosis) causes a broad and bifid P wave.

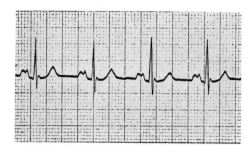

ABNORMALITIES OF THE QRS COMPLEX

The origins of small Q waves, and of R and S waves, were discussed in chapter 1. We now have to consider why the QRS complex should sometimes become unusually wide or unusually tall, and why big Q waves can develop.

1   Widening of the QRS

The width, or duration, of the QRS complex is determined by the time taken for the whole of the septum and ventricular muscle mass to be depolarised. If depolarisation spreads through the normal pathway the process is completed within 0·12 seconds (three small squares). If the depolarisation wave spreads by an abnormal route—as is necessary if some part of the special conducting tissue is damaged— then depolarisation takes longer, and the QRS is widened.

If the cardiac pacemaker is supraventricular, and yet the QRS complex is 0·16 seconds (four small squares) or more in duration, then one of the two bundle branches must be blocked. (Remember that the QRS complex is also widened in a ventricular extrasystole, again because of the abnormal, and slow, path of the depolarisation wave.) If both bundle branches are blocked, then there is complete heart block with 'ventricular escape'.

Right bundle branch block (RBBB) often indicates problems in the right side of the heart, but RBBB patterns with a normal duration of   the QRS complex are quite common in healthy people. Left bundle branch block (LBBB) is always an indication of heart disease, usually of the left side. It is important to recognise that bundle branch block is present, for LBBB prevents any further interpretation of the

47

cardiogram, and RBBB can make interpretation difficult.

The mechanism underlying the E.C.G. patterns of right and left bundle branch block can be worked out from first principles. Remember (chapter 1):

(a) The septum is normally depolarised from left to right.

(b) The left ventricle, having the greater muscle mass, exerts more influence on the E.C.G. than the right ventricle.

(c) Excitation spreading towards an electrode causes an upward deflection of the E.C.G.

Right bundle branch block. No conduction occurs down the right bundle branch, but the septum is depolarised from the left side as usual, causing an R wave in a right ventricular lead (V1) and a small Q in a left ventricular lead (V6).

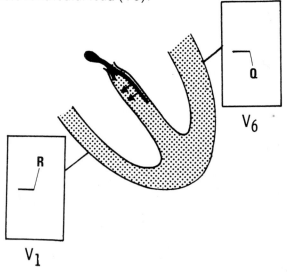

Excitation then spreads to the left ventricle, causing an S in V1 and an R in V6.

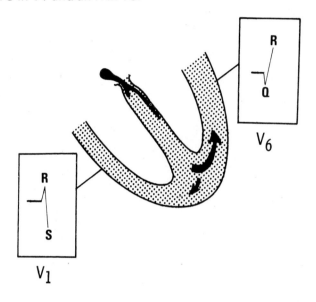

It takes longer for excitation to reach the right ventricle because of the failure of the normal conducting pathway, and the right ventricle therefore depolarises after the left. So there is a second R wave (R1) in V1, and a wide and deep S in V6.

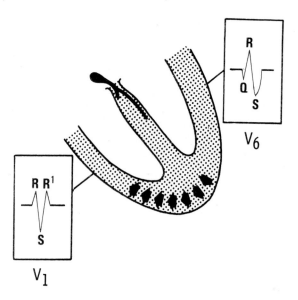

Abnormalities of the P, QRS, and T Waves

Left bundle branch block. If conduction down the left bundle branch fails, the septum has to be depolarised from right to left, causing a small Q in V1, and an R in V6.

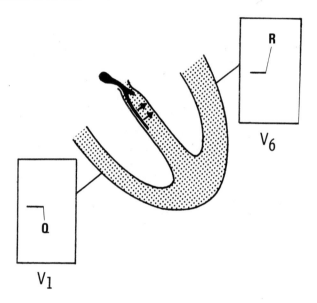

The right ventricle is depolarised before the left, so despite the smaller muscle mass there is an R in V1 and an S (often appearing only as a notch) in V6.

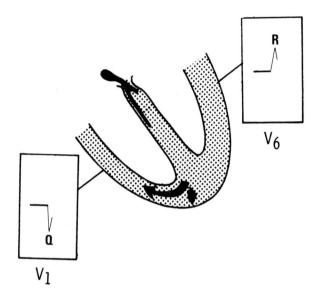

Later depolarisation of the left ventricle causes an S in V1 and another R in V6.

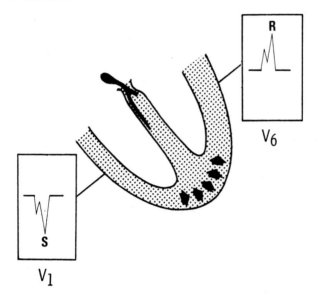

53

What to remember
RBBB is best seen in V1, where there is an RSR pattern.

RIGHT BUNDLE BRANCH BLOCK

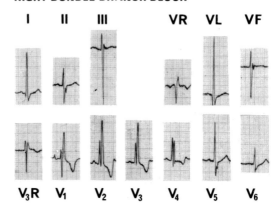

I II III VR VL VF

V₃R V₁ V₂ V₃ V₄ V₅ V₆

LBBB is best seen in V6, where there is an M pattern.

LEFT BUNDLE BRANCH BLOCK

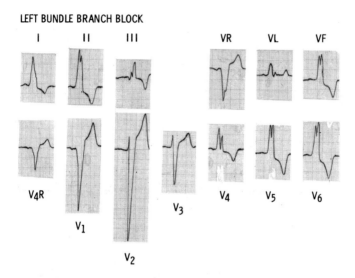

LBBB always means heart disease, and prevents any further interpretation of the E.C.G. RBBB, at least when 'partial' (QRS 0·12 seconds or less) *may* be seen in normal people, and it makes further interpretation difficult.

2   Increased height of the QRS complex

An increase of muscle mass in any part of the heart will lead to increased electrical activity, and to an increase in the height of the QRS complex.

Right ventricular hypertrophy is best seen in the right ventricular leads (especially V1), where the complex becomes upright (i.e. the height of the R wave exceeds the depth of the S)—this is always abnormal. There will be a deep S in V6.

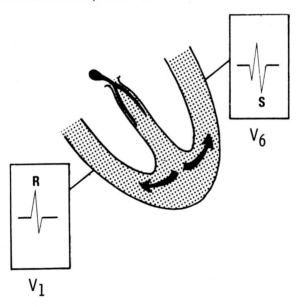

This is usually accompanied by right axis deviation
(chapter 1), by a peaked P wave (right atrial
hypertrophy), and in severe cases by inversion of the
T waves in V2 and V3.

RV HYPERTROPHY

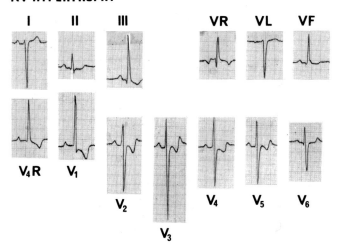

Left ventricular hypertrophy causes a tall R wave (greater than 25 mm in V5 or V6) and a deep S in V1 or V2—but in practice such 'voltage' changes alone are unhelpful in diagnosing left ventricular enlargement With significant hypertrophy there are also inverted T waves in V5 and V6, and there may be left axis deviation.

LV HYPERTROPHY

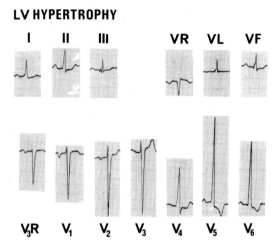

3   The Origin of Q waves

Small ('septal') Q waves in the left ventricular leads result from depolarisation of the septum from left to right (chapter 1). Q waves greater than 0·04 seconds (one small square) in duration, and greater than 2 mm (two small squares) in depth have, however, a quite different significance.

The ventricles are depolarised from inside outwards. Therefore an electrode placed in the cavity of the ventricle would record only a Q wave, as all the depolarisation waves would be moving away from it. If a myocardial infarction causes complete death of muscle from the inside surface to the outside surface of the heart, an electrical 'window' is created, and an electrode looking at the heart over that window will record a cavity potential—that is, a Q wave.

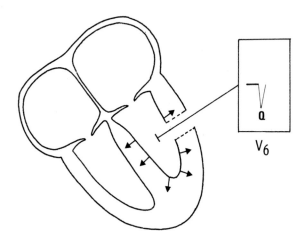

V_6

Q waves greater than one small square across and/or more than 2 mm deep therefore indicate a myocardial infarction, and the leads in which the Q wave appears give some indication of the part of the heart that has been damaged. Thus, infarction of the anterior wall of the left ventricle causes a Q wave in the leads looking at the heart from the front—V3, 4, 5 (chapter 1).

ANTERIOR INFARCTION

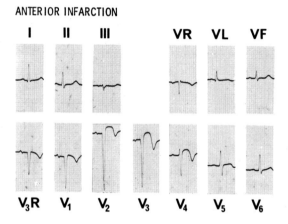

Abnormalities of the P, QRS, and T Waves

Infarctions of the inferior surface of the heart cause Q waves in the leads looking at the heart from below— III and VF.

INFERIOR INFARCTION

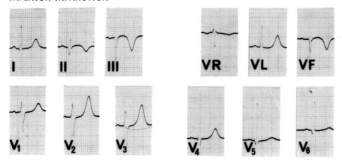

The presence of a Q wave does not, however, give any indication of the age of the infarction, for once a Q wave has developed it is usually permanent.

ABNORMALITIES OF THE ST SEGMENT

The ST segment lies between the QRS complex and the T wave.

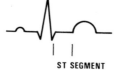

ST SEGMENT

It should be 'isoelectric'—that is, at the same level as the part between the T and the next P—but it may be elevated,

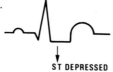

ST ELEVATED

or depressed.

ST DEPRESSED

Elevation of the ST segment is an indication of acute myocardial injury, usually due either to a recent infarction or to pericarditis. Again, the leads in which it occurs indicate the part of the heart that is damaged—anterior damage shows in the V leads, and inferior in III and VF. Pericarditis is not usually a localised affair, and therefore it causes ST elevation in most leads.

Abnormalities of the P, QRS, and T Waves

Horizontal depression of the ST segment, in association with an upright T wave, is usually a sign of ischaemia as opposed to infarction. When the E.C.G. at rest is normal, ST segment depression may appear on effort, particularly when effort induces angina.

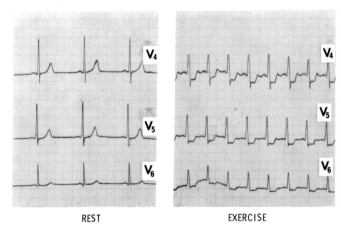

REST   EXERCISE

ABNORMALITIES OF THE T WAVE

The T wave may be lengthened or made taller by electrolyte (especially potassium) abnormalities: the most important change to look for is the lengthening to more than 0·4 seconds of the interval from the Q wave to the end of the T wave that accompanies low plasma potassium—this change may occur during diuretic therapy.

The most common abnormality is inversion of the T wave, which is seen in the following circumstances:

1   Normality. The T wave is normally inverted in VR and in V1 (and in V2 in young people, and also in V3 in Negroes).

63

2   Ischaemia. After a myocardial infarction the first
abnormality seen on the E.C.G. is elevation of the
ST segment. Subsequently Q waves appear, and
the T wave becomes inverted. The ST segment
returns to the baseline, the whole process
taking a variable time but usually 24 to 48
hours. T wave inversion is often permanent.

Chest pain for 6 hours

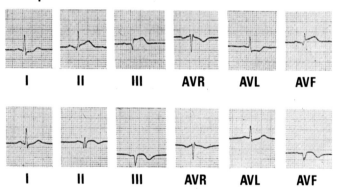

| I | II | III | AVR | AVL | AVF |

24 hours later

3   Ventricular hypertrophy. Left ventricular
hypertrophy causes inverted T waves in leads
looking at the left ventricle (V5, V6, II and
VL). (See above.) Right ventricular hypertrophy
causes T wave inversion in the leads looking at the
right ventricle (T inversion is normal in V1 but in
white adults not in V2 or V3).

4   Bundle branch block. The abnormal path of
depolarisation in bundle branch block is usually
associated with an abnormal path of repolarisation.

Therefore inverted T waves associated with QRS complexes 0·16 seconds or more in duration have no significance of themselves.

5   Digoxin. The administration of Digoxin causes T inversion, particularly with sloping depression of the ST segment. It is helpful to record an E.C.G. *before* beginning digitalis to save later confusion about the significance of T wave changes.

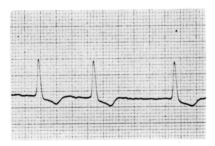

6   Non-specific changes. Minor degrees of ST segment and T wave abnormalities (T wave flattening, etc.) are usually of no great significance, and are best reported as 'non-specific ST–T changes'.

Things to remember

1 Tall P waves result from right atrial hypertrophy, and broad P waves from left atrial hypertrophy.
2 Broadening of the QRS complex indicates abnormal intraventricular conduction: it is seen in bundle branch block and in complexes originating in the ventricular muscle.
3 Increased height of the QRS complex indicates ventricular hypertrophy. Right ventricular hypertrophy is seen in V1, and left ventricular hypertrophy is seen in V5 and V6.
4 Q waves greater than 1 mm across and 2 mm deep indicate myocardial infarction.
5 ST segment elevation indicates acute myocardial infarction or pericarditis.
6 ST segment depression and T wave inversion may be due to ischaemia, ventricular hypertrophy abnormal intraventricular conduction, or digitalis.

CONCLUSIONS

1 The E.C.G. is easy to understand.
2 Most abnormalities of the E.C.G. are amenable to reason.

INDEX

Notes

Notes

Notes

Notes